Super Simple Slow Cooker Delicacies

Cheap and Easy On a Budget Recipes To Burn Fat and Save Time

Britney Cooke

© **Copyright 2020 - All rights reserved.**

The content contained within this book may not be reproduced, duplicated or transmitted without direct written permission from the author or the publisher.

Under no circumstances will any blame or legal responsibility be held against the publisher, or author, for any damages, reparation, or monetary loss due to the information contained within this book. Either directly or indirectly.

Legal Notice:

This book is copyright protected. This book is only for personal use. You cannot amend, distribute, sell, use, quote or paraphrase any part, or the content within this book, without the consent of the author or publisher.

Disclaimer Notice:

Please note the information contained within this document is for educational and entertainment purposes only. All effort has been executed to present accurate, up to date, and reliable, complete information. No warranties of any kind are declared or implied. Readers acknowledge that the author is not engaging in the rendering of legal, financial, medical or professional advice. The content within this book has been derived from various sources. Please consult a licensed professional before attempting any techniques outlined in this book.

By reading this document, the reader agrees that under no circumstances is the author responsible for any losses, direct or indirect, which are incurred as a result of the use of information contained within this document, including, but not limited to, — errors, omissions, or inaccuracies.

Table of contents

Black Bean Mushroom Chili 7
Caveman Chili 9
Perfect Eggplant Tapenade 11
Swiss Style Cheese Fondue 12
Tex-Mex Cheese Dip 14
Ingredient Cheese Dip 15
Asparagus Bacon Bouquet 16
Creamy Asiago Spinach Dip 17
Madras Curry Chicken Bites 19
Ranch Chicken 21
Sesame Ginger Chicken 22
Chicken Bacon Chowder 24
Chicken Lo Mein 26
Chicken with Bacon Gravy 28
Pizza Chicken 30
Green Beans & Chicken Thighs 31
Cheesy Adobo Chicken 33
Salmon with Lemon and Caper Sauce 35
Spicy BBQ Shrimp 37
Dill, Halibut, and Lemon 39
Cilantro Curry Shrimp 41
Shrimp with Marinara Sauce 43
Shrimp with Garlic 45
Poach Salmon 47
Lemon-Pepper Tilapia 49

Zoodles with Cauliflower-Tomato Sauce 51
Spaghetti Squash Carbonara 53
Summery Bell Pepper + Eggplant Salad 55
Butter Green Peas 56
Lemon Asparagus 57
Lime Green Beans 58
Cheese Asparagus 59
Creamy Broccoli 60
Garlic Eggplant 61
Coconut Brussels Sprouts 62
Cauliflower Pilaf with Hazelnuts 63
Cauliflower and Turmeric Mash 65
Kale Mash with Blue Cheese 66
Marinated Fennel Bulb 67
Zucchini Slices with Mozzarella 68
Pesto Spaghetti Squash 69
Grated Zucchini with Cheese 71
Cauliflower Croquettes 72
Cauliflower Puree with Parmesan 73
Red Cabbage Slices 74
Green Bean and Avocado Salad 75
Vegan Cauliflower Rice and Beans 77
Broccoli Mix 79
Roasted Beets 80
Lemony Pumpkin Wedges 81
Thai Side Salad 82
Eggplants with Mayo Sauce 83

Summer Squash Medley	85
Garlic Butter Green Beans	86
Green Beans and Red Peppers	87
Swedish Pea and Ham Soup	88
Fisherman's Stew	89
Seafood Gumbo	91
White Bean Soup with Shrimp	93
Crab and Corn Soup	95
Butternut Squash Soup with Parsnips	97
Serrano Pepper and Black Bean Soup	99
Sweet Potato Soup	101
Hot and Sour Soup	102
Peanut Soup (African Style)	104
Slow Cooker Pierogie Casserole	106
Spinach Noodle Casserole	108

Black Bean Mushroom Chili

Preparation Time: 17 Minutes

Cooking Time: 8 Hours and 25 Minutes

Servings: 10

Ingredients:

- 2 1/2 cups black beans, rinsed and drained
- 1 tbsp. olive oil
- 2 tbsp. chili powder
- 1/4 cup mustard seeds
- 1/2 tsp. cardamom seeds
- 1 1/2 tsp. cumin seeds
- 1/4 cup water
- 1 lb. mushrooms, sliced
- 2 onions, chopped
- 5 cups vegetable stock
- 1 tbsp. chipotle pepper in adobo sauce, chopped
- 6 oz. tomato paste
- 1 cup cheddar cheese, grated
- 1/2 cup sour cream
- 1/2 fresh cilantro, chopped

Directions:

1. Soak black beans overnight. Rinse and drain the next day.

2. Place oil, chili powder, mustard, cardamom, and cumin in a Dutch oven.
3. Cook over high heat for 30 seconds.
4. Add water, mushrooms, and onions.
5. Cover and cook for 7 minutes. Add broth, chipotles, and tomato paste.
6. Cook for another 15 minutes.
7. Put the beans in a slow cooker.
8. Add the vegetable mixture. Cook on high for 8 hours.
9. Garnish with sour cream, cilantro, and cheese before serving. Enjoy!

Nutrition: Calories 216, Fat 10, Carbs 13, Protein 10

Caveman Chili

Preparation Time: 20 Minutes

Cooking Time: 6 Hours and 15 Minutes

Servings: 8

Ingredients:
- 2 pounds ground pork
- 8 thick slices bacon, chopped
- 1 onion, chopped
- 3 small green bell peppers, chopped
- 1 (6 ounce) can tomato paste
- garlic powder
- Salt
- Cayenne pepper

Directions:

1. In a frying pan, put the pork over medium heat, then sprinkle with pepper and salt. Let it cook and stir for about 5-7 minutes, until it becomes crumbly and brown. Drain and get rid of the grease. Move the pork to a slow cooker.

2. In the hot frying pan, put the bacon and let it cook for about 10 minutes on medium-high heat until browned evenly. Drain and get rid of the grease. Move the bacon to the slow cooker.

3. In the slow cooker, mix the tomato paste, green bell pepper, onion, and drained tomatoes, then add the cayenne pepper, pepper, salt, onion powder, garlic powder, and seasoning packet. Mix to incorporate.

4. Let it cook for approximately 6 hours on low, until the flavors have blended.

Nutrition: Calories 336, Fat 22, Carbs 12, Protein 18

Perfect Eggplant Tapenade

Preparation time: 15 minutes

Cooking time: 9 hours

Servings: 2

Ingredients

- cups eggplants, chopped
- 1 cup tomatoes, chopped
- garlic cloves, minced
- 2 teaspoons capers
- 2 teaspoons fresh lemon juice
- 1 teaspoon dried basil
- Salt, to taste
- Pinch of ground black pepper

Directions:

1. In a slow cooker, add eggplant, tomatoes, garlic, and capers and mix well.
2. Cook on low, covered, for about 7-9 hours.
3. Uncover the slow cooker and stir in the remaining Ingredients
4. Serve hot.

Nutrition: Calories: 46 Carbohydrates: 10.1g Protein: 2g Fat: 0.4g Sugar: 5g Sodium: 170mgFiber: 4.2g

Swiss Style Cheese Fondue

Preparation time: 15 minutes

Cooking time: 3 hours & 10 minutes

Servings: 6

Ingredients

- 1 clove garlic, cut in half
- 2½ cups homemade chicken broth
- tablespoons fresh lemon juice
- 16 ounces' Swiss cheese, shredded
- ounces Cheddar cheese, shredded
- tablespoons almond flour
- Pinch of ground nutmeg
- Pinch of paprika
- Pinch of ground black pepper

Directions:

1. Rub a pan evenly with cut garlic halves. Add broth and place pan over medium heat.
2. Cook until mixture is just beginning to bubble. Adjust to low, then stir in lemon juice.
3. Meanwhile, in a bowl, mix cheeses and flour. Slowly, add cheese mixture to broth, stirring continuously.
4. Cook until cheese mixture becomes thick, stirring continuously. Transfer the cheese mixture to a

greased crockpot and sprinkle with nutmeg, paprika, and black pepper.

5   Cook in the slow cooker on low, covered, for about 1-3 hours.

Nutrition: Calories: 479 Carbohydrates: 6.1g Protein: 32.6g Fat: 36g Sugar: 1.8g Sodium: 700mg Fiber: 0.5g

Tex-Mex Cheese Dip

Preparation time: 15 minutes

Cooking time: 1 hour & 30 minutes

Servings: 6

Ingredients

- ounces Velveeta cheese, cubed
- ¾ cup diced tomatoes with green chili peppers
- 1 teaspoon taco seasoning

Directions:

1. In a slow cooker, place Velveeta cheese cubes.
2. Cook on low and cook, covered, for about 30-60 minutes, stirring occasionally.
3. Uncover the slow cooker and stir in tomatoes and taco seasoning. Cook, covered, for about 30 minutes
4. Serve hot.

Nutrition: Calories: 114 Carbohydrates: 5.2g Protein: 7g Fat: 8.1g Sugar: 3.4g Sodium: 577mg Fiber: 0.3g

Ingredient Cheese Dip

Preparation time: 15 minutes

Cooking time: 2 hours

Servings: 20

Ingredients

- 16 ounces Velveeta cheese, cubed
- 1 (16-ounce) jar salsa

Directions:

1. In a large slow cooker, place cheese and salsa and stir gently to combine.
2. Cook on high, covered, for about 2 hours, stirring occasionally. Serve hot.

Nutrition: Calories: 71 Carbohydrates: 3.9g Protein: 4.4g Fat: 4.9g Sugar: 2.3g Sodium: 460mg Fiber: 0.4g

Asparagus Bacon Bouquet

Preparation time: 15 minutes

Cooking time: 4 hours

Servings: 4

Ingredients

- asparagus spears, trimmed
- slices bacon
- 1 tsp black pepper
- Extra virgin olive oil

Directions:

1. Coat slow cooker with extra virgin olive oil.
2. Slice spears in half, and sprinkle with black pepper
3. Wrap three spear halves with one slice bacon, and set inside the slow cooker.
4. Cook for 4 hours on medium.

Nutrition: Calories 345 Carbs 2 g Fat 27 g Protein 22 g Sodium 1311 mg Sugar 0 g

Creamy Asiago Spinach Dip

Preparation time: 15 minutes

Cooking time: 4 hours

Servings: 6

Ingredients

- cups spinach, wash, chopped
- ½ cup artichoke hearts
- ½ cup cream cheese
- ½ cup Asiago cheese, grated
- ½ cup almond milk
- 1 tsp black pepper
- Extra virgin olive oil

Directions:

1. Coat slow cooker with olive oil.
2. Place cream cheese and almond milk in a blender, and mix until smooth.
3. Finely chop spinach, add to blender along with salt and black pepper, and mix.
4. Place spinach mixture in a blender, add artichoke hearts and mix in with a spatula.
5. Sprinkle Asiago cheese on top, and cook on medium for 4 hours.
6. Serve dip with a selection of veggies like broccoli florets and carrot sticks.

Nutrition: Calories 214 Carbs 4 g Fat 19 g Protein 8 g Sodium 380 mg Sugar 1 g

Madras Curry Chicken Bites

Preparation time: 15 minutes

Cooking time: 7 hours

Servings: 4

Ingredients

- 1 lb. chicken breasts, skinless, boneless
- cloves garlic, grated
- 1 tsp ginger, grated
- 2 cups low-sodium chicken stock
- 2 lemons, juiced
- 1 tsp coriander, crushed
- 1 tsp cumin
- ½ tsp fenugreek
- 1 tbsp. curry powder
- ½ tsp cinnamon
- 1½ tsp salt
- 1 tsp black pepper
- Extra virgin olive oil

Directions:

1. Cube chicken breast into ½" pieces, and sprinkle with ½ tsp salt and ½ tsp black pepper.
2. Heat 3 tbsp. extra virgin olive oil in a skillet, add chicken breasts, and brown.
3. Place chicken breasts in a slow cooker.

4   Add chicken stock, garlic, lemon juice, spices, and salt.
5   Cook on low for 7 hours.

Nutrition: Calories 234 Carbs 3 g Fat 8 g Protein 38 g Sodium 782 mg Sugar 0 g

Ranch Chicken

Preparation time : 5 minutes

Cooking time: 7 hours

Servings: 4 people

Slow cooker size: 6-quart

Ingredients:

- 2 pounds' skinless pasture-raised chicken breast
- 3 tablespoons dried ranch dressing
- 3 tablespoons butter, chopped
- 4-ounce cream cheese, chopped

Directions:

1. Place chicken in a 6-quart slow cooker, scatter with butter and cream cheese, and sprinkle with ranch dressing.
2. Shut with lid, then plug in the slow cooker and cook for 4 hours at high heat setting or 5 to 7 hours at low heat setting or until cooked. Shred chicken with two forks and stirs until evenly coated and serve straightaway.

Nutrition: Calories: 251.3 Fat: 12.9g Protein: 33g Carbs: 0.8g

Sesame Ginger Chicken

Preparation time: 5 minutes
Cooking time: 6 hours
Servings: 4 people

Slow cooker size: 6-quart

Ingredients:

- 1 ½ pound skinless pasture-raised chicken breasts
- 2 tablespoons chopped red bell pepper
- ¼ cup minced onion
- 1 teaspoon minced garlic
- ½ tablespoon grated fresh ginger
- ½ teaspoon crushed red pepper flakes
- 1 tablespoon swerve sweetener
- 2 tablespoons coconut aminos
- 3 tablespoons sesame seed oil
- ½ cup tomato puree
- 1/3 cup peach jam, sugar-free
- 1/3 cup chicken broth
- 2 teaspoons sesame seeds

Directions:

1. Place all the fixings in a 6-quart slow cooker, except for sesame seeds, chicken, and pepper, and stir until mixed.
2. Add chicken, turn to coat chicken with sauce and then top with red bell pepper. Plugin the slow

cooker, shut with lid, and cook for 6 hours at low heat setting or 4 hours at high heat setting. Garnish with sesame seeds and serve.

Nutrition: Calories: 180 Fat: 12.8g Protein: 37.8g Carbs: 2g

Chicken Bacon Chowder

Preparation time: 5 minutes

Cooking time: 9 hours & 5 minutes

Servings: 4 people

Slow cooker size : 6-quart

Ingredients:

- 1-pound pasture-raised chicken breast, skinless
- 1-pound bacon
- 6-ounce Cremini mushrooms
- 2 celeries, diced
- 1 medium white onion, peeled and diced
- 2 teaspoons minced garlic
- 1 teaspoon garlic powder
- 1 teaspoon salt
- 1 teaspoon ground black pepper
- 1 teaspoon dried thyme
- 2 tablespoons avocado oil
- 2 tablespoons unsalted butter
- 2 cups chicken stock
- 8-ounce cream cheese, cubed
- 1 cup heavy cream

Directions:

1. Plug in a 6-quart slow cooker and let preheat at a low heat setting. Then add mushrooms, celery,

onion, garlic, salt, black pepper, butter, and 1 cup stock and stir until mixed.

2. Shut with lid and cook for 1 hour at a low heat setting. Place a large skillet pan over medium-high heat, add oil and when hot, add oil and when hot, put the chicken and cook within 5 minutes or until seared on all sides.
3. Transfer seared chicken to a plate, deglaze the pan with remaining stock and stir well to remove browned bits stuck on the pan's bottom, and then add to slow cooker when vegetables are cooked.
4. Add remaining ingredients to cooked vegetables, stir well until cream cheese is mixed. Cut chicken into cubes, add to slow cooker along with bacon, and stir until mixed.
5. Shut with lid and cook for 6 to 8 hours at a low heat setting or until cooked. Serve.

Nutrition: Calories: 879.3 Fat: 66.4g Protein: 59.3g Carbs: 11g

Chicken Lo Mein

Preparation time: 15 minutes

Cooking time: 4 hours & 10 minutes

Servings: 4 people

Slow cooker size: 6-quart

Ingredients:

- 1 1/2 pounds' boneless pasture-raised chicken thighs, sliced
- 12 ounces' kelp noodles
- 1 bunch bok choy, sliced
- 1 teaspoon minced garlic
- 1 teaspoon grated ginger
- 1 ½ teaspoon salt
- ¾ teaspoon ground black pepper
- For Chicken Marinade:
- 1/2 teaspoon minced garlic
- 1 tablespoon coconut aminos
- 1/2 teaspoon avocado oil
- For Sauce:
- 1/2 teaspoon xanthan gum
- 1 tablespoon swerve sweetener
- 1 teaspoon red pepper chili flakes
- 1/4 cup coconut aminos
- 2 teaspoon sesame oil
- 1 tablespoon apple cider vinegar

- 3/4 cup chicken broth

Directions:

1. Place the ingredients for the marinade in a large bowl, whisk until combined, then add chicken, toss until well coated, and let marinate in the refrigerator for 30 minutes.
2. Then grease a 6-quart slow cooker with oil, add marinated chicken, and shut with lid. Cook within 2 hours at a low heat setting or for 1 hour at high heat.
3. Move the cooked chicken to a serving plate and add cabbage, ginger, garlic to the slow cooker, and top with chicken.
4. Whisk the sauce ingredients in a bowl, pour all over the chicken, and shut with lid—Cook for 1 hour to 2 hours on low or 30 minutes to 1 hour on high.
5. In the meantime, rinse kelp noodles and soak them in water. When cooking time is up, add kelp noodles to the slow cooker and stir with tongs until evenly coated with sauce.
6. Stir in xanthan gum and cook for 10 to 15 minutes on high. Serve straight away.

Nutrition: Calories: 198 Fat: 10.1g Protein: 24.5g Carbs: 3.1g

Chicken with Bacon Gravy

Preparation time: 5 minutes

Cooking time: 3 hours & 30 minutes

Servings: 4 people

Slow cooker size: 4-quart

Ingredients:

- 1 ½ pound skinless pasture-raised chicken breasts
- 6 slices of bacon, cooked and crumbled
- 1 teaspoon minced garlic
- ¼ teaspoon ground black pepper
- 1 teaspoon dried thyme
- 3 ½ tablespoons dried chicken gravy mix
- 4 tablespoons oil
- 1 ¼ cup of water
- 1 cup heavy cream

Directions:

1. Put chicken in a 4-quart slow cooker, add bacon and sprinkle with garlic, black pepper, and garlic, and drizzle with oil.
2. Whisk together water and chicken gravy mix until smooth, and then pour this mixture over the chicken.
3. Plugin the slow cooker, shut with lid, and cook for 3 ½ hours at a high heat setting or until chicken is cooked.

4. When done, add cream, then shred chicken with 2 forks and stir until well combined. Serve straight away.

Nutrition: Calories: 551 Fat: 38g Protein: 51g Carbs: 1.3g

Pizza Chicken

Preparation time : 5 minutes

Cooking time: 3 hours & 30 minutes

Servings: 4 people

Slow cooker size: 6-quart

Ingredients:

- 4 skinless pasture-raised chicken breasts
- 20 slices of pepperoni
- 1 ½ teaspoon salt
- 1 teaspoon ground black pepper
- 2 cups marinara sauce, sugar-free
- 1 cup grated parmesan cheese

Directions :

1. Spread marinara sauce into a 6-quart slow cooker, then add chicken and season with salt and black pepper. Plugin the slow cooker, top chicken with pepperoni slices, and shut with lid.
2. Cook chicken for 3 hours at a low heat setting, then add cheese and continue cooking for 15 to 30 minutes. Serve straight away.

Nutrition: Calories: 418 Fat: 20g Protein: 49g Carbs: 10.5g

Green Beans & Chicken Thighs

Preparation time: 5 minutes

Cooking time: 8 hours

Servings: 4 people

Slow cooker size: 6-quart

Ingredients:

- 4 skin-on pasture-raised chicken thighs
- 1-pound green beans, trimmed
- 2 large tomatoes, diced
- 1 medium white onion, peeled and diced
- 1 teaspoon minced garlic
- 2 teaspoons salt and more for seasoning chicken
- 1 teaspoon ground black pepper and more for seasoning chicken
- 1/4 cup fresh chopped dill
- 6 tablespoons avocado oil, divided
- 1 lemon, juiced
- 1 cup chicken broth
- 1 cup sour cream

Directions:

1. Place green beans in a 6-quarts slow cooker, add remaining ingredients except 3 tablespoons oil, chicken, and sour cream and stir until mixed.

2. Plugin slow cooker, top green beans with chicken, drizzle with oil, season with salt and black pepper, and shut with lid.
3. Cook for 8 hours at a low heat setting or 4 hours at a high heat setting or until chicken is cooked through. Serve with sour cream.

Nutrition: Calories: 622 Fat: 46.3g Protein: 35.7g Carbs: 15.5g

Cheesy Adobo Chicken

Preparation time: 5 minutes

Cooking time: 8 hours & 5 minutes

Servings: 4 people

Slow cooker size: 6-quart

Ingredients:

- 1-pound pasture-raised chicken breasts, skin on
- 2 tablespoons adobo sauce
- 1/2 cup salsa, sugar-free
- For Cheese Sauce:
- 1 tablespoon arrowroot powder
- 1 tablespoon unsalted butter
- 1/2 cup coconut milk, unsweetened and full-fat
- 6 tablespoons grated cheddar cheese
- 6 tablespoons grated Monterey jack cheese

Directions:

1. Place adobo sauce and salsa in a 6-quart slow cooker, whisk together until combined, and then add chicken.
2. Plugin the slow cooker, shut with lid and cook for 6 to 8 hours at low heat setting or 3 to 4 hours at high heat setting or until cooked. Shred chicken with two forks and tosses until mixed with the sauce.
3. Prepare cheese sauce and for this, place a medium saucepan over medium-high heat, add butter and

when it melts, whisk in arrowroot powder and simmer for 1 minute.
4. Then slowly whisk in milk until smooth and cook for 4 minutes or until sauce thickens slightly. Remove saucepan from heat, add cheese and stir well until cheese melts and the smooth sauce comes together. Pour cheese over chicken and serve.

Nutrition: Calories: 313 Fat: 21g Protein: 26g Carbs: 5g

Salmon with Lemon and Caper Sauce

Preparation Time: 5 Minutes

Cooking Time: 1 Hour and 30 Minutes

Servings: 4

Ingredients:

- 1 pound wild-caught salmon fillet
- 2 teaspoon capers, rinsed and mashed
- 1 teaspoon minced garlic
- 1 teaspoon salt
- ½ teaspoon ground black pepper
- 1/2 teaspoon dried oregano
- 1 teaspoon lemon zest
- 2 tablespoons lemon juice
- 4 tablespoons unsalted butter

Directions:

1. Cut salmon into four pieces, then season with salt and black pepper and sprinkle lemon zest on top.
2. Line a 6-quart slow cooker with parchment paper, place seasoned salmon pieces on it, and shut with lid.
3. Plug in the slow cooker and cook for 1 hour and 30 minutes or until salmon is cooked through.

4. When 10 minutes of cooking time is left, prepare lemon-caper sauce and for this, place a small saucepan over low heat, add butter and let it melt.

5. Then add capers, garlic, lemon juice, stir until mixed, and simmer for 1 minute.

6. Remove saucepan from heat and stir in oregano.

7. When salmon is cooked, spoon lemon-caper sauce on it and serve.

Nutrition: Net Carbs: 2.4g; Calories: 368.5; Total Fat: 26.6g; Saturated Fat: 10.1g; Protein: 19.5g; Carbs: 2.7g; Fiber: 0.3g; Sugar: 2g

Spicy BBQ Shrimp

Preparation Time: 5 Minutes

Cooking Time: 1 Hour and 30 Minutes

Servings: 6

Ingredients:

- 1 1/2 pounds large wild-caught shrimp, unpeeled
- 1 green onion, chopped
- 1 teaspoon minced garlic
- 1 ½ teaspoon salt
- ¾ teaspoon ground black pepper
- 1 teaspoon Cajun seasoning
- 1 tablespoon hot pepper sauce
- ¼ cup Worcestershire Sauce
- 1 lemon, juiced
- 2 tablespoons avocado oil
- 1/2 cup unsalted butter, chopped

Directions:

1. Place all the ingredients except for shrimps in a 6-quart slow cooker and whisk until mixed.
2. Plug in the slow cooker then shut with lid and cook for 30 minutes at a high heat setting.
3. Then take out ½ cup of this sauce and reserve.
4. Add shrimps to slow cooker.

Nutrition: Net Carbs: 2.4g; Calories: 321; Total Fat: 21.4g; Saturated Fat: 10.6g; Protein: 27.3g; Carbs: 4.8g; Fiber: 2.4g; Sugar: 1.2g

Dill, Halibut, and Lemon

Preparation Time: 5 Minutes

Cooking Time: 2 Hours

Servings: 2

Ingredients:

- 12-ounce wild-caught halibut fillet
- 1 teaspoon salt
- ½ teaspoon ground black pepper
- 1 1/2 teaspoon dried dill
- 1 tablespoon fresh lemon juice
- 3 tablespoons avocado oil

Directions:

1. Cut an 18-inch piece of aluminum foil, place halibut fillet in the middle and then season with salt and black pepper.
2. Whisk together remaining ingredients, drizzle this mixture over halibut, then crimp the edges of foil and place it into a 6-quart slow cooker.
3. Plug in the slow cooker, shut with lid, and cook for 1 hour and 30 minutes or 2 hours at high heat setting or until cooked through.
4. When done, carefully open the crimped edges and check the fish. It should be tender and flaky.

5. Serve straight away.

Nutrition: Net Carbs: 0g; Calories: 321.5; Total Fat: 21.4g; Saturated Fat: 7.2g; Protein: 32.1g; Carbs: 0g; Fiber: 0g; Sugar: 0.6g

Cilantro Curry Shrimp

Preparation Time: 5 Minutes

Cooking Time: 2 Hours and 30 Minutes

Servings: 4

Ingredients:

- 1 pound wild-caught shrimp, peeled and deveined
- 2 ½ teaspoon lemon garlic seasoning
- 2 tablespoons red curry paste
- 4 tablespoons chopped cilantro
- 30 ounces coconut milk, unsweetened
- 16 ounces of water

Directions:

1. Whisk together all the ingredients except for shrimps and two tablespoons cilantro and add to a 4-quart slow cooker.

2. Plug in the slow cooker, shut with lid, and cook for 2 hours at high heat setting or 4 hours at low heat setting.

3. Then add shrimps, toss until evenly coated and cook for 20 to 30 minutes at high heat settings or until shrimps are pink.

4. Garnish shrimps with remaining cilantro and serve.

Nutrition: Net Carbs: 1.9g; Calories: 160.7; Total Fat: 8.2g; Saturated Fat: 8.1g; Protein: 19.3g; Carbs: 2.4g; Fiber: 0.5g; Sugar: 1.4g

Shrimp with Marinara Sauce

Preparation Time: 5 Minutes

Cooking Time: 5 Hours and 10 Minutes

Servings: 5

Ingredients:

- 1 pound cooked wild-caught shrimps, peeled and deveined
- 14.5-ounce crushed tomatoes
- ½ teaspoon minced garlic
- 1 teaspoon salt
- 1/2 teaspoon seasoned salt
- ¼ teaspoon ground black pepper
- ½ teaspoon crushed red pepper flakes
- 1/2 teaspoon dried basil
- 1/2 teaspoon dried oregano
- ½ tablespoons avocado oil
- 6-ounce chicken broth
- 2 tablespoon minced parsley
- 1/2cupgratedParmesancheese

Directions:

1. Place all the ingredients except for shrimps, parsley, and cheese in a 4-quart slow cooker and stir well.

2. Then plug in the slow cooker, shut with lid, and cook for 4 to 5 hours at low heat setting.
3. Then add shrimps and parsley, stir until mixed and cook for 10 minutes at high heat setting.
4. Garnish shrimps with cheese and serve.

Nutrition: Net Carbs: 5.7g; Calories: 358.8; Total Fat: 25.1g; Saturated Fat: 4.3g; Protein: 26g; Carbs: 7.2g; Fiber: 1.5g; Sugar: 3.6g

Shrimp with Garlic

Preparation Time: 5 Minutes

Cooking Time: 60 Minutes

Servings: 5

Ingredients:

- For the Garlic Shrimp:
- 1 1/2 pounds large wild-caught shrimp, peeled and deveined
- 1/4 teaspoon ground black pepper
- 1/8 teaspoon ground cayenne pepper
- 2 ½ teaspoons minced garlic
- 1/4 cup avocado oil
- 4 tablespoons unsalted butter
- For the Seasoning:
- 1 teaspoon onion powder
- 1 tablespoon garlic powder
- 1 tablespoon salt
- 2 teaspoons ground black pepper
- 1 tablespoon paprika
- 1 teaspoon cayenne pepper
- 1 teaspoon dried oregano
- 1 teaspoon dried thyme

Directions:

1. Stir together all the ingredients for seasoning, garlic, oil, and butter and add to a 4-quart slow cooker.
2. Plug in the slow cooker, shut with lid, and cook for 25 to 30 minutes at high heat setting or until cooked.
3. Then add shrimps, toss until evenly coated, and continue cooking for 20 to 30 minutes at high heat setting or until shrimps are pink.
4. When done, transfer shrimps to a serving plate, top with sauce, and serve.

Nutrition: Net Carbs: 1.2g; Calories: 233.6; Total Fat: 11.7g; Saturated Fat: 1.3g; Protein: 30.9g; Carbs: 1.2g; Fiber: 0g; Sugar: 0g

Poach Salmon

Preparation Time: 5 Minutes

Cooking Time: 3 Hours and 35 Minutes

Servings: 4

Ingredients:

- 4 steaks of wild-caught salmon
- 1 medium white onion, peeled and sliced
- 2 teaspoons minced garlic
- 1/2 teaspoon salt
- 1/8 teaspoon ground white pepper
- 1/2 teaspoon dried dill weed
- 2 tablespoons avocado oil
- 2 tablespoons unsalted butter
- 2 tablespoons lemon juice
- 1 cup of water

Directions:

1. Place butter in a 4-quart slow cooker, then adds salmon and drizzle with oil.
2. Place remaining ingredients in a medium saucepan, stir until mixed and bring the mixture to boil over high heat.
3. Then pour this mixture all over salmon and shut with lid.

4. Plug in the slow cooker and cook salmon for 3 hours and 30 minutes at low heat setting or until salmon is tender.

5. Serve straight away.

Nutrition: Net Carbs: 2.8g; Calories: 310; Total Fat: 20g; Saturated Fat: 4.8g; Protein: 30.2g; Carbs: 3.1g; Fiber: 0.3g; Sugar: 1.2g

Lemon-Pepper Tilapia

Preparation Time: 5 Minutes

Cooking Time: 3 Hours

Servings: 6

Ingredients:

- 6 wild-caught Tilapia fillets
- 4 teaspoons lemon-pepper seasoning, divided
- 6 tablespoons unsalted butter, divided
- 1/2 cup lemon juice, fresh

Directions:

1. Cut a large piece of aluminum foil for each fillet and then arrange them on clean working space.
2. Place each fillet in the middle of the foil, then season with lemon-pepper seasoning, drizzle with lemon juice, and top with one tablespoon butter.
3. Gently crimp the edges of foil to form a packet and place it into a 6-quart slow cooker.
4. Plug in the slow cooker, shut with lid, and cook for 3 hours at high heat setting or until cooked through.

5. When done, carefully remove packets from the slow cooker and open the crimped edges and check the fish. It should be tender and flaky.
6. Serve straight away.

Nutrition: Net Carbs: 1.2 g; Calories: 201.2; Total Fat: 12.9g; Saturated Fat: 9.1g; Protein: 19.6g; Carbs: 1.5g; Fiber: 0.3g; Sugar: 0.7g

Zoodles with Cauliflower-Tomato Sauce

Preparation time: 15 minutes

Cooking time: 3 hours & 31 minutes

Servings: 4

Ingredients

- 5 large spiralized zucchinis
- Two 24-ounce cans of diced tomatoes
- 2 small heads' worth of cauliflower florets
- 1 cup chopped sweet onion
- 4 minced garlic cloves
- ½ cup veggie broth
- 5 teaspoons Italian seasoning
- Salt and pepper to taste
- Enough water to cover zoodles

Directions:

1. Put everything but the zoodles into your slow cooker. Cook on high for 3 ½ hours.
2. Smash into a chunky sauce with a potato masher or another utensil.
3. To cook the zoodles, boil a large pot of water. When boiling, cook zoodles for just 1 minute, then drain— Season with salt and pepper. Serve sauce over zoodles!

Nutrition: Calories: 113 Protein: 7g Carbs: 22g Fat: 2g Fiber: 10.5g

Spaghetti Squash Carbonara

Preparation time: 15 minutes

Cooking time: 8 hours & 10 minutes

Servings: 4

Ingredients

- 2 cups of water
- One 3-pound spaghetti squash
- ½ cup coconut bacon
- ½ cup fresh spinach leaves
- 1 egg
- 3 tablespoons heavy cream
- 3 tablespoons unsweetened almond milk
- ½ cup grated Parmesan cheese
- 1 teaspoon garlic powder
- Salt and pepper to taste

Directions:

1. Put squash in your cooker and pour in 2 cups of water. Close the lid.
2. Cook on low for 8-9 hours. When the spaghetti squash cools, mix egg, cream, milk, and cheese in a bowl.
3. When the squash is cool enough for you to handle with oven mitts, cut it open lengthwise and scrape out noodles. Mix in the egg mixture right away.

4. Add spinach and seasonings. Top with coconut bacon and enjoy!

Nutrition: Calories: 211 Protein: 5g Carbs: 26g Fat: 11g Fiber: 5.1g

Summery Bell Pepper + Eggplant Salad

Preparation time: 15 minutes

Cooking time: 7 hours

Servings: 4

Ingredients

- One 24-ounce can of whole tomatoes
- 2 sliced yellow bell peppers
- 2 small eggplants (smaller ones tend to be less bitter)
- 1 sliced red onion
- 1 tablespoon paprika
- 2 teaspoons cumin
- Salt and pepper to taste
- A squeeze of lime juice

Directions:

1. Mix all the fixings in your slow cooker. Close the lid. Cook on low for 7-8 hours.
2. When time is up, serve warm, or chill in the fridge for a few hours before eating.

Nutrition: Calories: 128 Protein: 5g Carbs: 27g Fat: 1g Fiber: 9.7g

Butter Green Peas

Preparation time: 10 minutes

Cooking time: 3 hours

Servings: 4

Ingredients

- 1 cup green peas
- 1 teaspoon minced garlic
- 1 tablespoon butter, softened
- ½ teaspoon cayenne pepper
- 1 tablespoon olive oil
- ¾ teaspoon salt
- 1 teaspoon paprika
- 1 teaspoon garam masala
- ½ cup chicken stock

Directions:

1. In the slow cooker, mix the peas with butter, garlic and the other **Ingredients:**
2. Close the lid and cook for 3 hours on High.

Nutrition: Calories 121, Fat 6.5, Fiber 3, Carbs 3.4, Protein 0.6

Lemon Asparagus

Preparation time: 8 minutes

Cooking time: 5 hours

Servings: 2

Ingredients

- 8 oz. asparagus
- ½ cup butter
- juice of 1 lemon
- Zest of 1 lemon, grated
- ½ teaspoon turmeric
- 1 teaspoon rosemary, dried

Directions:

1. In your slow cooker, mix the asparagus with butter, lemon juice and the other Ingredients: and close the lid.
2. Cook the vegetables on Low for 5 hours. Divide between plates and serve.

Nutrition: Calories 139, Fat 4.6., Fiber 2.5, Carbs 3.3, Protein 3.5

Lime Green Beans

Preparation time: 10 minutes

Cooking time: 2.5 hours

Servings: 5

Ingredients

- 1-pound green beans, trimmed and halved
- 2 spring onions, chopped
- 2 tablespoons lime juice
- ½ teaspoon lime zest, grated
- 2 tablespoons olive oil
- ¼ teaspoon ground black pepper
- ¾ teaspoon salt
- ¾ cup of water

Directions:

1. In the slow cooker, mix the green beans with the spring onions and the other **Ingredients:** and close the lid.
2. Cook for 2.5 hours on High.

Nutrition: Calories 67, Fat 5.6, Fiber 2, Carbs 4, Protein 2.1

Cheese Asparagus

Preparation time: 10 minutes

Cooking time: 3 hours

Servings: 4

Ingredients

- 10 oz. asparagus, trimmed
- 4 oz. Cheddar cheese, sliced
- 1/3 cup butter, soft
- 1 teaspoon turmeric powder
- ½ teaspoon salt
- ¼ teaspoon white pepper

Directions:

1. In the slow cooker, mix the asparagus with butter and the other Ingredients, put the lid on and cook for 3 hours on High.

Nutrition: Calories 214, Fat 6.2, Fiber 1.7, Carbs 3.6, Protein 4.2

Creamy Broccoli

Preparation time: 15 minutes

Cooking time: 1 hour

Servings: 4

Ingredients

- ½ cup coconut cream
- 2 cups broccoli florets
- 1 teaspoon mint, dried
- 1 teaspoon garam masala
- 1 teaspoon salt
- 1 tablespoon almonds flakes
- ½ teaspoon turmeric

Directions:

1. In the slow cooker, mix the broccoli with the mint and the other Ingredients.
2. Close the lid and cook vegetables for 1 hour on High.
3. Divide between plates and serve.

Nutrition: Calories 102, Fat 9, Fiber 1.9, Carbs 4.3, Protein 2.5

Garlic Eggplant

Preparation time: 15 minutes

Cooking time: 2 hours

Servings: 4

Ingredients

- 1-pound eggplant, trimmed and roughly cubed
- 1 tablespoon balsamic vinegar
- 1 garlic clove, diced
- 1 teaspoon tarragon
- 1 teaspoon salt
- 1 tablespoon olive oil
- ½ teaspoon ground paprika
- ¼ cup of water

Directions:

1. In the slow cooker, mix the eggplant with the vinegar, garlic and the other Ingredients, close the lid and cook on High for 2 hours.
2. Divide into bowls and serve.

Nutrition: Calories 132, Fat 2.8, Fiber 4.7, Carbs 8.5, Protein 1.6

Coconut Brussels Sprouts

Preparation time: 10 minutes

Cooking time: 4 hours

Servings: 6

Ingredients

- 2 cups Brussels sprouts, halved
- ½ cup of coconut milk
- 1 teaspoon garlic powder
- 1 teaspoon salt
- ½ teaspoon coriander, ground
- 1 teaspoon dried oregano
- 1 tablespoon balsamic vinegar
- 1 teaspoon butter

Directions:

1. Place Brussels sprouts in the slow cooker.
2. Add the rest of the Ingredients, toss, close the lid and cook the Brussels sprouts for 4 hours on Low.
3. Divide between plates and serve.

Nutrition: Calories 128, Fat 5.6, Fiber 1.7, Carbs 4.4, Protein 3.6

Cauliflower Pilaf with Hazelnuts

Preparation time: 15 minutes

Cooking time: 2 hours

Servings: 6

Ingredients

- 3 cups cauliflower, chopped
- 1 cup chicken stock
- 1 teaspoon ground black pepper
- ½ teaspoon turmeric
- ½ teaspoon ground paprika
- 1 teaspoon salt
- 1 tablespoon dried dill
- 1 tablespoon butter
- 2 tablespoons hazelnuts, chopped

Directions:

1. Put cauliflower in the blender and blend until you get cauliflower rice.
2. Then transfer the cauliflower rice in the slow cooker.
3. Add ground black pepper, turmeric, ground paprika, salt, dried dill, and butter.
4. Mix up the cauliflower rice. Add chicken stock and close the lid.

5. Cook the pilaf for 2 hours on High.

6. Then add chopped hazelnuts and mix the pilaf well.

Nutrition: Calories 48, Fat 3.1, Fiber 1.9, Carbs 4.8, Protein 1.6

Cauliflower and Turmeric Mash

Preparation time: 10 minutes

Cooking time: 3 hours

Servings: 3

Ingredients

- 1 cup cauliflower florets
- 1 teaspoon turmeric powder
- 1 cup of water
- 1 teaspoon salt
- 1 tablespoon butter
- 1 tablespoon coconut cream
- 1 teaspoon coriander, ground

Directions:

1. In the slow cooker, mix the cauliflower with water and salt.
2. Close the lid and cook for 3 hours on High.
3. Then drain water and transfer the cauliflower to a blender.
4. Add the rest of the Ingredients, blend and serve.

Nutrition: Calories 58, Fat 5.2, Fiber 1.2, Carbs 2.7, Protein 1.1

Kale Mash with Blue Cheese

Preparation Time: 15 Minutes

Cooking Time: 5 Hours

Servings: 3

Ingredients:

- 3 oz Blue cheese
- 1 cup Italian dark-leaf kale
- ¾ cup almond milk, unsweetened
- 1 tablespoon butter
- 1 teaspoon salt
- 1 teaspoon ground black pepper

Directions:

1. Chop the kale and place it in the slow cooker.
2. Add almond milk, salt, and ground black pepper.
3. Close the lid and cook the kale for 5 hours on Low.
4. Meanwhile, chop Blue cheese and butter.
5. Combine the cooked kale with the butter and stir it until butter is melted.
6. Add the Blue cheese and stir it gently.
7. Serve!

Nutrition: Calories 285, Fat 26.3, Fiber 1.8, Carbs 6.8, Protein 8.2

Marinated Fennel Bulb

Preparation Time: 10 Minutes

Cooking Time: 4 Hours

Servings: 2

Ingredients:

- 8 oz fennel bulb
- 1 tablespoon apple cider vinegar
- 1 garlic clove, diced
- 1 teaspoon dried oregano
- 5 tablespoons almond milk, unsweetened
- 1 teaspoon butter

Directions:

1. Chop the fennel bulb roughly and sprinkle it with the apple cider vinegar, diced garlic clove, and dried oregano.
2. Stir and let marinate for 15 minutes.
3. Place the chopped fennel in the slow cooker.
4. Add butter and almond milk.
5. Close the lid then cook it for 4 hours on Low.
6. Then chill the cooked fennel slightly and serve!

Nutrition: Calories 144, Fat 11.2, Fiber 4.7, Carbs 11.4, Protein 2.5

Zucchini Slices with Mozzarella

Preparation Time: 15 Minutes

Cooking Time: 1 Hour

Servings: 4

Ingredients:

- 3 oz Mozzarella, sliced
- 1 zucchini, sliced
- 1 tablespoon olive oil
- 1 teaspoon butter
- 1 tablespoon coconut flakes, unsweetened
- 1 teaspoon minced garlic

Directions:

1. Sprinkle the zucchini slices with the olive oil, coconut flakes, and minced garlic.
2. Place the zucchini slices in a flat layer on the bottom of the slow cooker along with the butter.
3. Place a piece of mozzarella on top of each zucchini slice.
4. Close the lid and cook the meal for 1 hour on High.
5. Serve hot!

Nutrition: Calories 112, Fat 8.7, Fiber 0.7, Carbs 2.8, Protein 6.7

Pesto Spaghetti Squash

Preparation Time: 15 Minutes

Cooking Time: 6 Hours

Servings: 4

Ingredients:

- 1 cup spinach
- 2 tablespoons olive oil
- 1 oz pumpkin seeds, crushed
- 1-pound spaghetti squash
- 1 teaspoon butter
- ¾ cup water

Directions:

1. Chop the spaghetti squash and put it in the slow cooker.
2. Add butter and water.
3. Close the lid and cook for 6 hours on Low.
4. Meanwhile, chop the spinach and place it in the blender.
5. Add olive oil and pumpkin seeds.
6. Blend the mixture until smooth.
7. When the spaghetti squash is cooked, transfer it into the serving bowls and sprinkle with the spinach (pesto) mixture.
8. Serve it!

Nutrition: Calories 144, Fat 11.9, Fiber 0.5, Carbs 9.4, Protein 2.7

Grated Zucchini with Cheese

Preparation Time: 15 Minutes

Cooking Time: 30 Minutes

Servings: 4

Ingredients:

- 2 oz Parmesan cheese, grated
- 1 zucchini, grated
- 1 teaspoon ground black pepper
- 1 tablespoon olive oil
- 1 teaspoon dried dill
- 4 tablespoons water

Directions:

1. Mix the grated zucchini, ground black pepper, and dried dill.
2. Stir the mixture and transfer it to the slow cooker.
3. Add water and olive oil.
4. Then sprinkle a layer of Parmesan cheese over the zucchini and close the lid.
5. Cook the meal for 30 minutes on High.
6. Serve the dish hot!

Nutrition: Calories 85, Fat 6.7, Fiber 0.7, Carbs 2.6, Protein 5.3

Cauliflower Croquettes

Preparation Time: 20 Minutes

Cooking Time: 2 Hours

Servings: 4

Ingredients:

- 1 egg
- 8 oz cauliflower, grated
- 1 teaspoon salt
- 3 tablespoons almond flour
- 1 tablespoon butter
- ½ teaspoon cayenne pepper

Directions:

1. Beat the egg in a bowl.
2. Add grated cauliflower, salt, and cayenne pepper to the whisked egg and stir.
3. Then make small balls from the mixture and coat them with the almond flour.
4. Toss the butter in the slow cooker.
5. Add the cauliflower croquettes to the slow cooker as well and cook them for 2 hours on High.
6. Let the cooked croquettes cool for at least 10 minutes.
7. Serve!

Nutrition: Calories 176, Fat 14.6, Fiber 3.7, Carbs 7.7, Protein 7.1

Cauliflower Puree with Parmesan

Preparation Time: 15 Minutes

Cooking Time: 6 Hours

Servings: 5

Ingredients:

- 1-pound cauliflower
- 1 cup water
- 2 tablespoons butter
- 2 oz Parmesan, grated

Directions:

1. Chop the cauliflower then put it in the slow cooker.
2. Add the water and close the lid.
3. Cook the cauliflower for 6 hours on Low.
4. Strain the cauliflower and place it in the blender.
5. Add the butter and blend it until you get a smooth puree.
6. Transfer the cauliflower puree to serving plates and sprinkle with grated Parmesan.
7. Serve it!

Nutrition: Calories 100, Fat 7.1, Fiber 2.3, Carbs 5.2, Protein 5.5

Red Cabbage Slices

Preparation Time: 15 Minutes

Cooking Time: 1 Hour

Servings: 4

Ingredients:

- 14 oz red cabbage
- 4 tablespoons olive oil
- 1 teaspoon dried oregano
- 1 teaspoon dried dill
- 4 tablespoons water
- 1 teaspoon salt

Directions:

1. Slice the red cabbage and sprinkle it with the olive oil, dried oregano, dried dill, and salt. Stir well.
2. Transfer the red cabbage mix into the slow cooker.
3. Add the water and close the lid.
4. Cook the red cabbage for 1 hour on High.
5. Serve the cabbage immediately!

Nutrition: Calories 147, Fat 14.2, Fiber 2.7, Carbs 6.1, Protein 1.4

Green Bean and Avocado Salad

Preparation Time: 15 Minutes

Cooking Time: 2 Hours

Servings: 4

Ingredients:

- 1 avocado, peeled, pitted
- 8 oz green beans
- 1 cup water
- 1 teaspoon ground black pepper
- 1 teaspoon salt
- 1 cucumber, chopped
- 1 teaspoon butter
- 1 oz walnuts, chopped
- 1 tablespoon olive oil

Directions:

1. Put the green beans in the slow cooker.
2. Add the water, ground black pepper, and salt.
3. Close the lid and cook the green beans for 2 hours on High.
4. Meanwhile, chop the avocado and put it in a salad bowl.
5. Add the chopped cucumber, walnuts, and olive oil to the salad bowl as well
6. Add the cooked warm green beans and stir the salad.

7. Enjoy it!

Nutrition: Calories 216, Fat 18.6, Fiber 6.3, Carbs 12.1, Protein 4.3

Vegan Cauliflower Rice and Beans

Preparation Time: 5 Minutes

Cooking Time: 4 Hours

Servings: 6

Ingredients:

- 24 oz cauliflower rice, frozen
- ½ cup hulled hemp seeds
- 1 cup vegetable stock
- 3 tbsp olive oil
- 2 tbsp garlic powder
- 1 tbsp onion powder
- 1 tbsp cumin
- 1 tbsp chili powder
- ½ tbsp cumin
- 1 tbsp chili powder
- ½ tbsp cayenne powder
- 1 tbsp Mexican oregano

Directions:

1. Add all the ingredients to the slow cooker except oregano, then stir well to mix.
2. Cover the slow cooker and cook on high for 4 hours. The rice should be tender.
3. Garnish as you desire, then serve. Enjoy.

Nutrition: Calories 278, Total Fat 20.2g, Saturated Fat 9g, Total Carbs 4.9g, Net Carbs 2.1g,

Protein 19.3g, Sugar: 2g, Fiber: 11.8g

Broccoli Mix

Preparation time: 15 minutes

Cooking time: 2 Hours

Servings: 10

Ingredients

- cups broccoli florets
- 1 and ½ cups cheddar cheese, shredded
- ounces canned cream of celery soup
- ½ teaspoon Worcestershire sauce
- ¼ cup yellow onion, chopped
- Salt and black pepper to the taste
- 1 cup crackers, crushed
- tablespoons soft butter

Directions:

1. In a bowl, mix broccoli with cream of celery soup, cheese, salt, pepper, onion and Worcestershire sauce, toss and transfer to your Crock Pot.
2. Add butter, toss again, sprinkle crackers, cover and cook on High for hours.
3. Serve as a side dish.

Nutrition: Calories 159, Fat 11, Fiber 1, Carbs 11, Protein 6

Roasted Beets

Preparation time: 15 minutes

Cooking time: 4 Hours

Servings: 5

Ingredients

- small beets
- teaspoons olive oil
- A pinch of salt and black pepper

Directions:

1. Divide each beet on a tin foil piece, drizzle oil, season them with salt and pepper, rub well, wrap beets, place them in your Crock Pot, cover and cook on High for 4 hours.
2. Unwrap beets, cool them down a bit, peel, and slice and serve them as a side dish.

Nutrition: Calories 100, Fat 2, Fiber 2, Carbs 4, Protein 5

Lemony Pumpkin Wedges

Preparation time: 15 minutes

Cooking time: 6 Hours

Servings: 4

Ingredients

- 15 oz. pumpkin, peeled and cut into wedges
- 1 tbsp. lemon juice
- 1 tsp. salt
- 1 tsp. honey
- ½ tsp. ground cardamom
- 1 tsp. lime juice

Directions:

1. Add pumpkin, lemon juice, honey, lime juice, cardamom, and salt to the Crock Pot.
2. Put the slow cooker's lid on and set the cooking time to 6 hours on Low settings.
3. Serve fresh.

Nutrition: Calories: 35, Total Fat: 0.1g, Fiber: 1g, Total Carbs: 8.91g, Protein: 1g

Thai Side Salad

Preparation time: 15 minutes
Cooking time: 3 Hours
Servings: 8

Ingredients

- ounces' yellow summer squash, peeled and roughly chopped
- ounces' zucchini, halved and sliced
- cups button mushrooms, quartered
- 1 red sweet potato, chopped
- leeks, sliced
- tablespoons veggie stock
- garlic cloves, minced
- tablespoon Thai red curry paste
- 1 tablespoon ginger, grated
- 1/3 cup coconut milk
- ¼ cup basil, chopped

Directions:

1. In your Crock Pot, mix zucchini with summer squash, mushrooms, red pepper, leeks, garlic, stock, curry paste, ginger, coconut milk and basil, toss, cover and cook on Low for 3 hours.
2. Stir your Thai mix one more time, divide between plates and serve as a side dish.

Nutrition: Calories 69, Fat 2, Fiber 2, Carbs 8, Protein 2

Eggplants with Mayo Sauce

Preparation time: 15 minutes

Cooking time: 5 Hours

Servings: 8

Ingredients

- tbsp. minced garlic
- 1 chili pepper, chopped
- 1 sweet pepper, chopped
- tbsp. mayo
- 1 tsp. olive oil
- 1 tsp. salt
- ½ tsp. ground black pepper
- 18 oz. eggplants, peeled and diced
- tbsp. sour cream

Directions:

1. Blend chili pepper, sweet peppers, salt, garlic, and black pepper in a blender until smooth.
2. Add eggplant and this chili mixture to the Crock Pot then toss them well.
3. Now mix mayo with sour cream and spread on top of eggplants.
4. Put the cooker's lid on and set the cooking time to 5 hours on High settings.
5. Serve warm

Nutrition: Calories: 40, Total Fat: 1.1g, Fiber: 3g, Total Carbs: 7.5g, Protein: 1g

Summer Squash Medley

Preparation time: 15 minutes

Cooking time: 2 hours

Servings: 4

Ingredients

- ¼ cup olive oil
- tbsp. basil, chopped
- tbsp. balsamic vinegar
- garlic cloves, minced
- tsp. mustard
- Salt and black pepper to the taste
- summer squash, sliced
- zucchinis, sliced

Directions:

1. Add squash, zucchinis, and all other **Ingredients:** to the Crock Pot.
2. Put the cooker's lid on and set the cooking time to hours on High settings.
3. Serve.

Nutrition: Calories: 179, Total Fat: 13g, Fiber: 2g, Total Carbs: 10g, Protein: 4g

Garlic Butter Green Beans

Preparation time: 15 minutes

Cooking time: 2 Hours

Servings: 6

Ingredients

- 22 ounces' green beans
- garlic cloves, minced
- ¼ cup butter, soft
- tablespoons parmesan, grated

Directions:

1. In your Crock Pot, mix green beans with garlic, butter and parmesan, toss, cover and cook on High for 2 hours.
2. Divide between plates, sprinkle parmesan all over and serve as a side dish.

Nutrition: Calories 60, Fat 4, Fiber 1, Carbs 3, Protein 1

Green Beans and Red Peppers

Preparation time: 15 minutes

Cooking time: 2 Hours

Servings: 2

Ingredients

- cups green beans, halved
- 1 red bell pepper, cut into strips
- Salt and black pepper to the taste
- 1 tablespoon olive oil
- 1 and ½ tablespoon honey mustard

Directions:

1. In your Crock Pot, mix green beans with bell pepper, salt, pepper, oil and honey mustard, toss, cover and cook on High for 2 hours.
2. Divide between plates and serve as a side dish.

Nutrition: Calories 50, Fat 0, Fiber 4, Carbs 8, Protein 2

Swedish Pea and Ham Soup

Preparation Time: 10 Minutes
Cooking Time: 5 Hours
Servings: 8

Ingredients:

- 3 cups yellow split peas, rinsed and drained
- 4 cups water
- 4 cups low sodium chicken stock
- 1 cup carrots, diced
- 2 cups onions, diced
- 1 tbsp. fresh ginger, minced
- 8 oz. ham, sliced
- 1 tsp. dried marjoram
- 1/4 tsp. pepper

Directions:

1. Put the split peas, water, stock, carrots, onions, celery, ginger, ham, and marjoram in the slow cooker.
2. Stir to blend everything. Put the lid on.
3. For 4 hours and 30 minutes to 5 hours, cook it on high.
4. Season with pepper before serving. Enjoy!

Nutrition: Calories 338, Fat 3, Carbs 23, Protein 21

Fisherman's Stew

Preparation Time: 17 Minutes

Cooking Time: 8 Hours and 35 Minutes

Servings: 6

Ingredients:

- 2 tbsp. olive oil
- 2 garlic cloves, finely chopped
- 1 cup baby carrots, sliced 1/4 inch thick
- 6 large Roma tomatoes, sliced and quartered
- 1 green bell pepper, chopped
- 1/2 tsp. fennel seed
- 1 cup water
- 1 bottle (8 oz.) clam juice
- 1-pound cod, cut into 1-inch cubes
- 1/2-pound medium shrimp, uncooked, peeled, and deveined
- 1 tsp. sugar
- 1 tsp. dried basil leaves
- 1/2 tsp. salt
- 1/4 tsp. red pepper sauce
- 2 tbsp. fresh parsley, chopped

Directions:

1. Stir the olive oil, garlic, carrots, tomatoes, green pepper, fennel seed, water, and clam juice together in the slow cooker.
2. Cover then cook it for 8 to 9 hours on LOW. Vegetables should be tender.
3. Twenty minutes before serving, add cod, shrimp, sugar, basil, salt, and pepper sauce.
4. Cover and cook 15 to 20 minutes on HIGH. The soup is ready when the fish can easily be flaked and shrimp are pink in color. Serve and enjoy!

Nutrition: Calories 180, Fat 26, Carbs 10, Protein 10

Seafood Gumbo

Preparation Time: 17 Minutes

Cooking Time: 2 Hours and 20 Minutes

Servings: 6

Ingredients:

- 8 to 10 bacon strips, sliced
- 2 stalks celery, sliced
- 1 medium onion, sliced
- 1 green pepper, chopped
- 2 garlic cloves, minced
- 2 cups chicken broth
- 1 can (14 oz.) diced tomatoes, undrained
- 2 tbsp. Worcestershire sauce
- 2 tsp. salt
- 1 tsp. dried thyme leaves
- 1-pound large raw shrimp, peeled, deveined
- 1 pound fresh or frozen crabmeat
- 1 box (10 oz.) frozen okra, thawed and sliced into 1/2-inch pieces

Directions:

1. Brown the bacon in a skillet through medium heat. When crisp, drain and transfer to a slow cooker.
2. Drain off drippings, leaving just enough to coat the skillet.

3. Sauté celery, onion, green pepper, and garlic until vegetables are tender.
4. Transfer the sautéed vegetables to the slow cooker.
5. Add the broth, tomatoes, Worcestershire sauce, salt, and thyme.
6. Cover then cook it for 4 hours on LOW, or for 2 hours on HIGH.
7. Add the shrimp, crabmeat, and okra. Cover and cook 1 hour longer on LOW or 30 minutes longer on HIGH. Serve and enjoy!

Nutrition: Calories 263, Fat 8, Carbs 13, Protein 4

White Bean Soup with Shrimp

Preparation Time: 15 Minutes

Cooking Time: 6 Hours and 15 Minutes

Servings: 8

Ingredients:

- 2 strips thick-cut bacon, unflavored
- 1 large onion, diced
- 2 garlic cloves, minced
- 1-pound kale, washed and roughly chopped
- 1 cup dried barley
- 1 1/2 cups dried navy beans
- 6 cups low sodium chicken broth
- 4 cups water
- 8 oz. cooked shrimp

Directions:

1. Brown the bacon in a skillet through a medium heat. When crisp, drain and transfer to slow cooker.
2. Drain off the drippings, leaving just enough to coat the skillet.
3. Sauté the onion and garlic until tender.
4. Transfer to a slow cooker.
5. Place kale, barley, and beans in the slow cooker.

6. Pour in the broth and water, and stir.
7. Cover and cook for 6-8 hours on LOW. Check occasionally to see if more water needs to be added.
8. About 20 minutes before the end of cooking, add the cooked shrimps and stir to heat through. Serve and enjoy!

Nutrition: Calories 149, Fat 3, Carbs 15, Protein 16

Crab and Corn Soup

Preparation Time: 17 Minutes

Cooking Time: 4 Hours and 10 Minutes

Servings: 6

Ingredients:

- 1-quart chicken stock
- 1 tbsp. butter or coconut butter
- 1 large onion, chopped
- 6 cups corn kernels, fresh or frozen
- 2 garlic cloves, chopped
- 1 tsp. salt
- 1/2 tsp. cayenne pepper
- 1 can (6 oz.) lump crabmeat, drained
- 1 cup half and half or coconut cream
- 1 avocado, cubed, for garnishing

Directions:

1. Place the chicken stock, butter, onion, corn kernels, garlic, salt, cayenne pepper, and crabmeat in the slow cooker.
2. Cover and cook for 4 hours on HIGH or 8 hours on LOW.
3. Blend with an immersion blender to get a smooth, thick consistency. (A regular blender may also be

used. Puree in small batches to prevent spillage. Be careful, liquid is hot! Remove lid insert to allow steam to escape.)

4. Stir in half and half or coconut cream.

5. Serve topped with avocado. Enjoy!

Nutrition: Calories 250, Fat 14, Carbs 25, Protein 5

Butternut Squash Soup with Parsnips

Preparation Time: 10 Minutes

Cooking Time: 6 Hours and 10 Minutes

Servings: 8

Ingredients:

- 1 large sweet onion, chopped
- 3 large parsnips, peeled and chopped
- 1 large Granny Smith apple
- 1/4 tsp. salt
- 1 tsp. freshly ground black pepper
- 3 cups water
- 2 cups chicken broth, low-sodium, fat-free
- 3 packages (12 oz.) frozen butternut squash, thawed
- 2 tbsp. whipping cream or coconut cream
- 1/8 tsp. paprika
- 1/8 tsp. ground cumin
- 1/2 cup light sour cream
- Chopped fresh chives (optional)

Directions:

1. Place the onion, parsnips, apple, salt, pepper, water, broth, and squash in the slow cooker. Stir.
2. Cover then cook it for 6 hours on LOW.

3. Puree using an immersion blender until smooth. (A regular blender may also be used. Puree in small batches to prevent spillage. Be careful, liquid is hot! Remove lid insert to allow steam to escape.)

4. Stir in the whipping cream, paprika, and cumin.

5. Serve and add a spoonful of sour cream on top, sprinkled with chives. Enjoy!

Nutrition: Calories 131, Fat 5, Carbs 13, Protein 4

Serrano Pepper and Black Bean Soup

Preparation Time: 10 Minutes

Cooking Time: 10 Hours and 15 Minutes

Servings: 6

Ingredients:

- 2 cups dried black beans, cleaned, soaked overnight, and drained
- 4 cups organic vegetable broth
- 2 onions, chopped
- 1 cup water
- 1 tbsp. ground cumin
- 3 bay leaves
- 1 serrano pepper, finely chopped
- 2 tbsp. fresh lime juice
- 1 tsp. salt
- 1/4 cup chopped fresh cilantro
- 3 tbsp. reduced-fat sour cream

Directions:

1. Combine the beans, broth, onions, water, cumin, bay leaves, and serrano pepper in the slow cooker.
2. Cover then cook it for 10 hours on LOW.

3. Remove the bay leaves, season with salt, and stir in lime juice.
4. Serve topped with sour cream and cilantro. Enjoy!

Nutrition: Calories 286, Fat 2, Carbs 23, Protein 17

Sweet Potato Soup

Preparation Time: 17 Minutes

Cooking Time: 3 Hours and 10 Minutes

Servings: 4

Ingredients:

- 2 sweet potatoes, peeled and diced
- 1/2 onion, minced
- Garlic
- Basil
- Salt and pepper

Directions:

1. Place all the fixings in a slow cooker and stir.
2. Cover and cook for 3 hours on HIGH. Puree with an immersion blender until the soup is smooth.
3. Serve and enjoy!

Nutrition: Calories 127, Fat 5, Carbs 1, Protein 20

Hot and Sour Soup

Preparation Time: 15 Minutes

Cooking Time: 8 Hours

Servings: 6

Ingredients:

- 1 package (10 oz.) packaged mushrooms, sliced
- 8 fresh shiitake mushroom caps, sliced
- 1 can (8 oz.) bamboo shoots, drained and julienned
- 4 garlic cloves, minced
- 1 package (15 oz.) tofu, cubed
- 2 tbsp. grated fresh ginger (divided)
- 4 cups water
- 2 tbsp. vegan chicken-flavored bouillon
- 2 tbsp. soy sauce
- 1 tsp. sesame oil
- 1 tsp. chili paste
- 2 tbsp. rice wine vinegar
- 1 1/2 cups peas, fresh or frozen

Directions:

1. Combine all the fixings in the slow cooker.
2. Cook for 6-8 hours on LOW. The mushrooms and bamboo shoots should be tender.
3. Add the peas and remaining 1 tablespoon ginger. Stir.

4. Adjust taste with vinegar or chili paste, if needed.

5. Serve with a few more drops of sesame oil and the chili paste on the side. Enjoy!

Nutrition: Calories 208, Fat 7, Carbs 22, Protein 19

Peanut Soup (African Style)

Preparation Time: 17 Minutes

Cooking Time: 6 Hours and 10 Minutes

Servings: 8

Ingredients:

- 1 yellow onion, diced
- 2 sprigs, chopped
- 2 red bell peppers, chopped
- 4 garlic cloves, minced
- 1 can (28 oz.) crushed tomatoes, undrained
- 8 cups vegetable broth
- 1/4 black pepper
- 1 tsp. ground cumin
- 1/4 tsp. chili powder
- 1/4 cup uncooked brown lentils
- 1/2 cup uncooked brown rice
- 1 cup peanut butter
- Sour cream and Tabasco sauce for topping

Directions:

1. Combine the onions, peppers, garlic, tomatoes, broth, black pepper, cumin, chili powder, lentils, and rice in the slow cooker.
2. Cover then cook it for 6-8 hours on LOW or 4 hours on HIGH. The onions should be translucent.

3. Stir in the butter and cook 30 minutes more on HIGH.

4. Serve topped with sour cream and Tabasco sauce. Enjoy!

Nutrition: Calories 245, Fat 7, Carbs 23, Protein 10

Slow Cooker Pierogie Casserole

Preparation Time: 15 Minutes

Cooking Time: 4 Hours

Servings: 4

Ingredients:

- 3 tablespoons butter
- 1 head cabbage, chopped
- 1 onion, chopped
- 1-pound bacon
- 4 (16.9 ounce) packages of frozen pierogies
- 3 tablespoons butter

Directions:

1. In a big pot, melt 3 tablespoons of butter over medium heat. Mix in onion and cabbage. Stir and cook for 20 minutes until the cabbage is soft.

2. In a big, deep frying pan, put bacon and cook over medium-high heat for 10 minutes until turning brown evenly, flipping sometimes. Put the bacon slices on a dish lined with paper towels to strain. Slice the bacon into bite-sized pieces and put aside.

3. Fully boil a big pot filled with lightly salted water over high heat. When the water boils, mix in

pierogies and boil again. Cook for 5 minutes until the pierogies rise to the surface; strain.

4. In a slow cooker, put the leftover 3 tablespoons of butter. Lightly mix bacon, cabbage, and pierogies; and put into the slow cooker. Cook for 3 hours on Low before eating.

Nutrition: Calories 579, Fat 18, Carbs 33, Protein 11

Spinach Noodle Casserole

Preparation Time: 15 Minutes

Cooking Time: 2 Hours

Servings: 5

Ingredients:

- 8 ounces' dry spinach noodles
- 2 tablespoons vegetable oil
- 1 1/2 cups sour cream
- 1/3 cup all-purpose flour
- 1 1/2 cups cottage cheese
- 4 green onions, minced
- 2 teaspoons Worcestershire sauce
- 1 dash hot pepper sauce
- 2 teaspoons garlic salt

Directions:

1. In a large pot, cook noodles in the salted boiling water until they are barely tender. Drain, then rinse under the cold water. Toss with the vegetable oil.

2. In a large bowl, combine flour and sour cream while the noodles are cooking. Mix well. Stir in garlic salt, hot pepper sauce, Worcestershire sauce, green onions, and cottage cheese. Stir the noodles into the mixture. Grease inside of the slow cooker generously. Pour in the noodle mixture.

3. Cook, covered, for 90-120 mins on high.

Nutrition: Calories 226, Fat 14, Carbs 14, Protein 8

Lightning Source UK Ltd.
Milton Keynes UK
UKHW021145040821
388300UK00013B/583